A BODYWORKER'S GUIDE TO

SOFT TISSUE PAIN PATTERNS

PRISCILLA FLEMING

DISCLAIMER

This book is intended to be an informational guide for licensed
bodyworkers. This book does not offer medical advice to the reader.
The information in this book is not intended to substitute professional
medical care or treatment. The remedies, corrective actions, and
techniques offered should not be used to treat a serious ailment
without prior consultation with a licensed physician.

INTRODUCTION

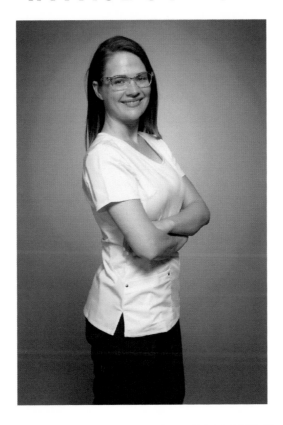

MY NAME IS PRISCILLA FLEMING. I AM A LICENSED MASSAGE THERAPIST CERTIFIED IN CLINICAL NEUROMUSCULAR THERAPY AND STRUCTURAL BODYWORK.

THIS BOOK IS INTENDED TO BE A QUICK REFERENCE GUIDE FOR LICENSED BODYWORKERS. THE SUGGESTED CORRECTIVE ACTIONS, CAUSATIVE FACTORS, AND SYMPTOMS ARE NOT AN EXHAUSTIVE LIST.

TABLE OF CONTENTS

LEG & FOOT

GASTROCNEMIUS — 02
"Calf Cramp Muscle"

SOLEUS — 03
"Joggers Heel" "Second Heart"

TIBIALIS POSTERIOR — 04
"Runner's Nemesis"

LONG FLEXORS OF THE TOES — 05
"Claw Toe or Hammer Toe Muscles"

POPLITEUS — 06
"Bent Knee Troublemaker"

TIBIALIS ANTERIOR — 07
"The Foot Drop Muscle"

PERONEUS (FIBULARIS) LONGUS/BREVIS — 08
"Weak Ankle Muscles"

EXTENSOR DIGITORUM LONGUS/EXTENSOR HALLICUS LONGUS — 09
"Hammer Toe Muscles"

PELVIS & THIGH

BICEPS FEMORIS — 11
"Chair Seat Victims"

SEMITENDINOSUS/ SEMIMEMBRANOSUS — 12
"Chair Seat Victims"

GLUTEUS MAXIMUS — 13
"Swimmer's Nemesis"

GLUTEUS MEDIUS — 14
"Lumbago Muscle"

GLUTEUS MINIMUS — 15
"Pseudo-Sciatica"

PIRIFORMIS + THE DEEP LATERAL ROTATORS — 16
"Double Devil"

RECTUS FEMORIS — 17
"Two Joint Puzzler"

VASTUS MEDIALIS — 18
"Buckling Knee Muscle"

PELVIS & THIGH (CONT.)

VASTUS INTERMEDIUS — 19
"The Frustrator"

VASTUS LATERALIS — 20
"Stuck Patella Muscle" "Nest of Hornets"

TENSOR FASCIAE LATAE — 21
"Pseudo-Trochanteric Bursitis"

SARTORIUS — 22
N/A

ADDUCTORS (MAGNUS, LONGUS, BREVIS — 23
"Obvious Problem Makers"

PECTINEUS — 24
"The Fourth Adductor"

GRACILIS — 25
N/A

ILIOPSOAS — 26
"The Hidden Prankster"

SPINE & THORAX

RECTUS ABDOMINIS + THE ABDOMINALS — 28
"The Limbo Limiters"

ERECTOR SPINAE — 29
N/A

SERRATUS POSTERIOR SUPERIOR/INFERIOR — 30
N/A

QUADRATUS LUMBORUM — 31
"The Joker of the Low Back"

TABLE OF CONTENTS

SHOULDER & ARM

PECTORALIS MAJOR — 33
"Chest & Shoulder Nuisance"

PECTORALIS MINOR — 34
"Thoracic Outlet Imposter"

SERRATUS ANTERIOR — 35
"Stitch in the Side Muscle"

SUPRASPINATUS — 36
"Overhead Activity Archenemy"

INFRASPINATUS — 37
"Side-Sleeper's Nemesis"

TERES MINOR — 38
"Infraspinatus' Little Brother" "Thrower's Trial"

SUBSCAPULARIS — 39
"Pseudo Frozen Shoulder Syndrome"

LATISSIMUS DORSI — 40
"Midback Manipulator"

TERES MAJOR — 41
"Lat's Little Brother" "Forgotten Shoulder Agitator"

RHOMBOIDS — 42
"Shoulder Blade Sorceres"

DELTOID — 43
"Overt Bothered"

BICEPS BRACHII — 44
N/A

BRACHIALIS — 45
"Beer Drinker's Muscle"

CORACOBRACHIALIS — 46
"Armpit Muscle"

TRICEPS BRACHII — 47
N/A

ANCONEUS — 48
N/A

FOREARM & HAND

SUPINATOR — 50
"The Tennis Elbow Muscle"

PRONATOR TERES — 51
N/A

FOREARM & HAND (CONT.)

BRACHIORADIALIS — 52
N/A

EXTENSORS OF THE FOREARM + WRIST — 53
N/A

FLEXORS OF THE FOREARM + WRIST — 54
N/A

HEAD, NECK, FACE

TRAPEZIUS — 56
"The Stress Headache Producer"

LEVATOR SCAPULAE — 57
"Crick in the Neck"

SPLENII - SPLENIUS CAPITIS + SPLENIUS CERVICIS — 58
N/A

SUBOCCIPITALS — 59
"The Bobble Head Muscles" "Ghostly Headache Muscles"

STERNOCLEIDOMASTOID (SCM) — 60
N/A

SCALENES (ANTERIOR, MIDDLE, POSTERIOR) — 61
N/A

DIGASTRIC — 62
"Pseudo SCM Pain"

ALL OTHER ANTERIOR NECK MUSCLES — 63

MUSCLES OF THE FACE — 64

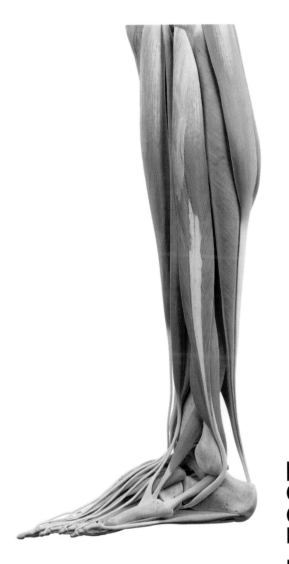

LEG & FOOT

GASTROCNEMIUS
"CALF CRAMP MUSCLE"

PAIN PATTERN

- Same side instep
- Medial ankle
- Back of calf up to posterior thigh
- Back of knee

SYMPTOMS

- Nocturnal calf cramps
- Localized calf pain without decreased range of motion or weakness

CAUSATIVE/PERPETUATING FACTORS

- Chronic plantar flexion
- High heels
- Driving
- Cycling
- Running
- Immobility of leg
- Reduced circulation into legs (tight sock elastic)
- Improper gait
- Excessive pronation

CORRECTIVE ACTIONS

- Stretch
- Sustained dorsiflexion
- Heel drops
- Lunges
- Active resisted stretching
- Moist heat

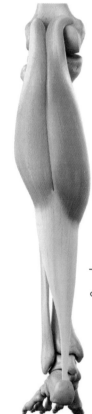

Posterior view
of left leg & foot

SOLEUS
"THE JOGGERS HEEL"
"SECOND HEART"

PAIN PATTERN

- Distal portion of soleus/Achilles
- Ipsilateral SI pain
- Proximal posterior calf

SYMPTOMS

- Heel pain
- Restricted dorsiflexion
- Limited ROM in talocrural joint
- Difficulty using stairs

CAUSATIVE/PERPETUATING FACTORS

- Chronic plantar flexion
- High heels
- Driving
- Inappropriate recovery after workout
- Cycling
- Reduced circulation into legs
- Bedridden
- Improper gait
- Excessive pronation
- Sudden overload/misstep
- Uneven or soft terrain (sand)

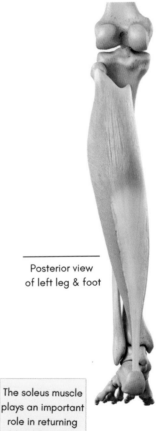

Posterior view
of left leg & foot

CORRECTIVE ACTIONS

- Stretch
- Sustained dorsiflexion
- Heel drops
- Lunges
- Active resisted stretching
- Moist heat

The soleus muscle plays an important role in returning blood from the legs.

04 TIBIALIS POSTERIOR
"RUNNER'S NEMESIS"

PAIN PATTERN

- Achilles tendon
- Spray over entire plantar surface

SYMPTOMS

- Pain when walking or running

CAUSATIVE/PERPETUATING FACTORS

- Chronic plantar flexion
- High heels
- Driving
- Inappropriate recovery after workout
- Cycling
- Reduced circulation into legs
- Bedridden
- Improper gait
- Excessive pronation
- Sudden overload/misstep
- Uneven or soft terrain (sand)
- Morton's foot
- Hammer toes

CORRECTIVE ACTIONS

- Stretch
- Sustained dorsiflexion
- Heel drops
- Lunges
- Active resisted stretching
- Moist heat

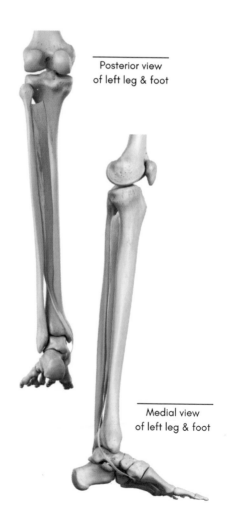

Posterior view
of left leg & foot

Medial view
of left leg & foot

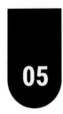
LONG FLEXORS OF THE TOES
"CLAW TOE OR HAMMER TOE MUSCLES"

PAIN PATTERN

- Big toe
- Plantar surface of 2nd-5th phalanges

CAUSATIVE/PERPETUATING FACTORS

- Chronic plantar flexion
- High heels
- Driving
- Inappropriate recovery after workout
- Cycling
- Reduced circulation into legs
- Bedridden
- Improper gait
- Excessive pronation
- Sudden overload/misstep
- Uneven or soft terrain (sand)
- Morton's foot
- Hammer toes

SYMPTOMS

- Pain in toes (if no toe pain, treat calf muscles)
- Claw/Hammer Toes

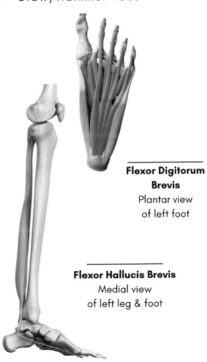

Flexor Digitorum Brevis
Plantar view
of left foot

Flexor Hallucis Brevis
Medial view
of left leg & foot

CORRECTIVE ACTIONS

- Stretch
- Sustained dorsiflexion
- Heel drops
- Lunges
- Active resisted stretching

CORRECTIVE ACTIONS (CONT.)

- Moist heat
- Towel/yoga strap stretch
- Stretch toes back during calf stretch

> Long flexors of the toes consist of Flexor digitorum longus/brevis & Flexor hallucis longus/brevis.

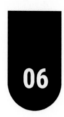

POPLITEUS
"BENT KNEE TROUBLEMAKER"

PAIN PATTERN

- Back of knee (localized pain)

CAUSATIVE/PERPETUATING FACTORS

- Abrupt stopping of femur during rapid lower body twist
- Soccer, football, skiing
- Plantaris tear
- Baker's cyst (contraindication)
- Knee gout (contraindication)
- Bursitis (contraindication)
- Jumping, cutting, cross fit box jumps

CORRECTIVE ACTIONS

- Calf/hamstring stretch
- Calf/hamstring release

SYMPTOMS

- Pain in back of knee while running, crouching, or walking downhill/down stairs
- Inability to straighten knee

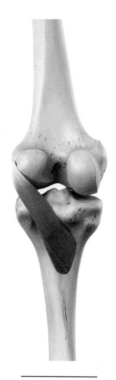

Posterior view
of left knee

TIBIALIS ANTERIOR
"THE FOOT DROP MUSCLE"

PAIN PATTERN

- Anterior medial aspect of ankle
- Dorsal and medial surface of great toe
- Shin down to ankle

CAUSATIVE/PERPETUATING FACTORS

- Overload in posterior compartment
- Walking on soft ground/slanted surface (running on curved road)
- Acute trauma
- Twisting ankles (rapid contraction during inversion)
- Tripping during contraction phase of walking - reflex response to sudden stretch
- Flip flops

CORRECTIVE ACTIONS

- Release calf muscle tightness
- Correct body mechanics/posture
- Morton's foot structure – refer out

SYMPTOMS

- Referred pain and tenderness in ankle
- Painful motion of ankle
- Dragging of toes/ankle weakness
- Tripping while walking
- May feel like symptoms of extensors
- Inflammation along tibia
- Tenderness, tightness goes around entire leg

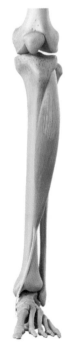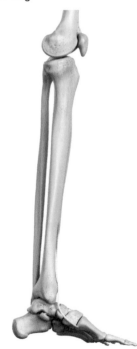

| Anterior view of left leg & foot | Medial view of left leg & foot |

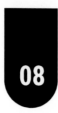

PERONEUS (FIBULARIS) LONGUS/ BREVIS

"WEAK ANKLE MUSCLES"

08

PAIN PATTERN

- Lateral malleolus
- Lateral aspect of foot
- Lateral aspect of middle third of leg

CAUSATIVE/PERPETUATING FACTORS

- Prolonged immobilization of leg/foot by cast
- Morton's foot structure
- Crossing legs while seated
- High heels
- Flat feet
- Tight elastic around calf
- Flip flops

CORRECTIVE ACTIONS

- Bring foot/ankle through ROM in warm water
- Moist heat
- Stretch

SYMPTOMS

- Pain in lateral ankle
- Ankle weakness
- Tendons can rupture spontaneously
- Nerve pain
- Sprain ankles frequently
- Vulnerable to fractures

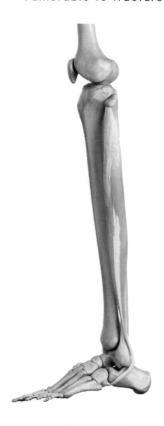

Lateral view
of left leg & foot

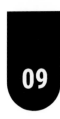

EXTENSOR DIGITORUM LONGUS/ EXTENSOR HALLICUS LONGUS
"HAMMER TOE MUSCLES"

PAIN PATTERN

- Digitorum: dorsolateral aspect of foot to tips of middle three toes
- Hallucis: dorsal aspect of foot to big toe
- Ankle
- Lower half of lower leg

CAUSATIVE/PERPETUATING FACTORS

- Acute stress overload
- Flip flops
- Walking in soft sand
- Excessive driving
- Prolonged plantar flexion
- Very tight gastrocnemius and soleus muscles

CORRECTIVE ACTIONS

- Halt excessive running or jogging
- Keep warm
- Avoid overstretching positions (high heels)
- Avoid flip flops

SYMPTOMS

- "Growing pains" in children
- Foot slap
- Hammer toes

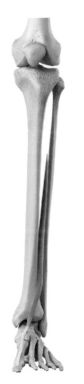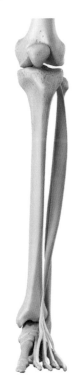

Extensor Hallucis Longus
Anterior view of left leg & foot

Extensor Digitorum Longus
Anterior view of left leg & foot

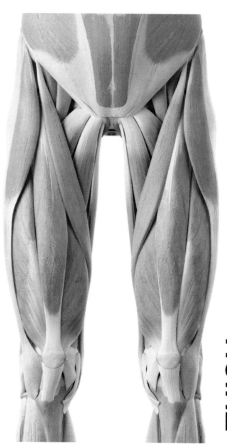

PELVIS & THIGH

BICEPS FEMORIS

"CHAIR SEAT VICTIMS"

PAIN PATTERN

- Back of the knee up lateral thigh to the crease of the buttocks

CAUSATIVE/PERPETUATING FACTORS

- Acute trauma from under-thigh pressure from a high-fitting edge of a chair
- Quadricep overload

SYMPTOMS

- Pain sitting and walking

CORRECTIVE ACTIONS

- Use pillow or cushion when seated
- Long seated reach exercise

Chair check –

When seated, your hand should slide between your thigh and the chair.

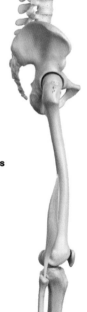

Short head of Biceps Femoris
Lateral view of right hip & thigh

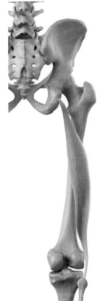

Long head of Biceps Femoris
Posterior view of right hip & thigh

SEMITENDINOSUS/ SEMIMEMBRANOSUS

"CHAIR SEAT VICTIMS"

PAIN PATTERN

- Lower buttocks to below the knee on the medial thigh

CAUSATIVE/PERPETUATING FACTORS

- Acute trauma from under-thigh pressure from a high-fitting edge of a chair
- Quadricep overload

SYMPTOMS

- Pain sitting and walking

CORRECTIVE ACTIONS

- Use pillow or cushion when seated
- Long seated reach exercise

Hamstring pain can be caused by eight other muscles besides hamstrings (satellite trigger points).

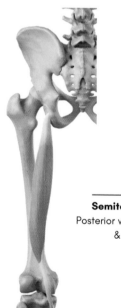

Semitendinosus
Posterior view of left hip & thigh

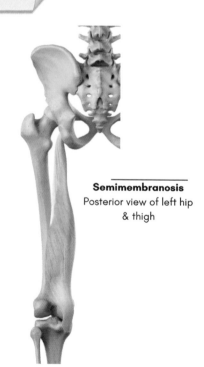

Semimembranosis
Posterior view of left hip & thigh

GLUTEUS MAXIMUS
"SWIMMER'S NEMESIS"

PAIN PATTERN

- At ischium, sacrum, ilium, sacrotuberous ligament, and greater tuberosity
- Localized muscle pain (hurts where it is)
- Attachment site pain
- Pain when sitting – sacrotuberous ligament

CAUSATIVE/PERPETUATING FACTORS

- Fall or near fall
- Impact trauma
- Swimming
- Sleeping incorrectly
- Morton's toe
- Pure body mechanics
- Prolonged walking in forward leaning position

CORRECTIVE ACTIONS

- Sitting on a cushion
- Sleeping with pillow between legs
- Stretch, hold, exhale, deeper stretch (repeat three times)
- Roll out on a tennis ball
- Get up and walk around when sitting for a long period of time

SYMPTOMS

- Restlessness
- Pain with sitting or climbing (hills, stairs)
- "Ants in your pants" (tingling sensation)
- Difficult time finding comfortable position
- Can affect ischial tuberosity (hamstring attachment)

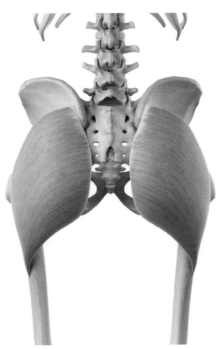

Posterior view

GLUTEUS MEDIUS
"LUMBAGO MUSCLE"
(LOW BACK PAIN)

PAIN PATTERN

- Ilium, sacrum, lumbar region of back
- Mid buttocks
- May extend into upper thigh
- When one side is overloaded, both sides of the sacrum can hurt

CAUSATIVE/PERPETUATING FACTORS

- Morton's foot structure
- Sitting on wallet
- Crossing legs while sitting
- Walking on uneven terrain (sand)
- Poor posture
- Near fall
- Extended sitting
- Running
- Weight bearing on one limb
- Carrying baby on hip

SYMPTOMS

- Difficulty sleeping on affected side (prolonged abduction)
- Pain while walking
- Uncomfortable sitting in slumped position

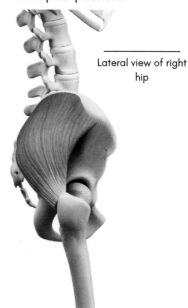

Lateral view of right hip

CORRECTIVE ACTIONS

- Stretch
- Roll out on tennis ball
- Sleep with pillow between legs
- Remove wallet from back pocket when seated

CORRECTIVE ACTIONS (CONT.)

- Refer out when necessary (if muscle treatment does not work)
- Recumbent bike to reactivate muscles (cannot prescribe exercises but can suggest changing angle of bike seat)

GLUTEUS MINIMUS
"PSEUDO-SCIATICA"

PAIN PATTERN

- Lateral thigh to ankle
- Knee
- Lower leg to the ankle
- Back of leg and thigh

CAUSATIVE/PERPETUATING FACTORS

- Prolonged immobility
- Sitting on wallet
- Fall or near fall
- Overuse in athletic activities
- Limping
- Wearing a boot/cast
- Morton's foot structure

CORRECTIVE ACTIONS

- Stretch
- Place pillow between knees while side lying/sleeping
- Ice
- Change position often

SYMPTOMS

- Pain when standing up from a chair
- Walking

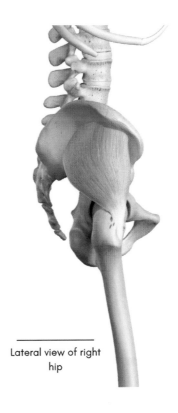

Lateral view of right hip

TIP:
Sit down to put pants on. balancing on one leg can overload the glute muscles.

PIRIFORMIS + THE DEEP LATERAL ROTATORS
"DOUBLE DEVIL" (PIRIFORMIS)

PAIN PATTERN

- Pain in SI region
- Buttocks
- Posterior hip joint
- Proximal two thirds of posterior thigh

CAUSATIVE/PERPETUATING FACTORS

- Sitting, standing, walking
- Acute overload
- Fall or near fall
- Running
- Holding thigh flexed in abduction (driving)

CORRECTIVE ACTIONS

- Correct functional leg length discrepancy
- Maintain correct sleep position
- Get out of car when driving for long periods of time
- Stretch
- Ischemic compression on trigger point – but avoid nerve (would not suggest tennis ball)

SYMPTOMS

- Nerve entrapment
- SI joint dysfunction

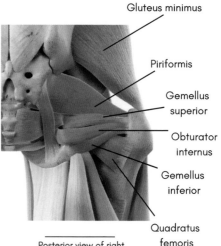

Gluteus minimus

Piriformis

Gemellus superior

Obturator internus

Gemellus inferior

Quadratus femoris

Posterior view of right hip

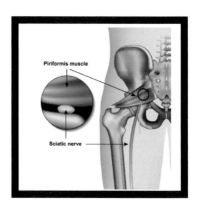

Piriformis muscle

Sciatic nerve

RECTUS FEMORIS
"TWO-JOINT PUZZLER"

PAIN PATTERN

- Anterior knee pain - deep pain/ache
- Most common trigger point is at the origin

SYMPTOMS

- May manifest at night
- Going down stairs is difficult
- No limits in range of motion
- No positional relief

CAUSATIVE/PERPETUATING FACTORS

- Sedentary lifestyle
- Chronic hip flexion - (sitting/driving/flying)
- Chronic kneeling
- Sudden overload through misstep or fall
- Excessively tight hamstrings
- Knee surgery
- Hiking/running downhill
- Hernia surgery

CORRECTIVE ACTIONS

- Quad stretch with extended hip (knee under client's knee)
- Heel to butt stretch (grab toes to create plantar flexion)
- Lunge, camel, pigeon, dancer pose stretches

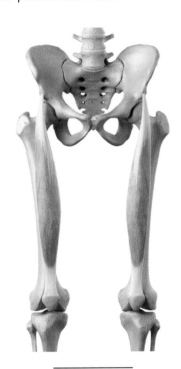

Anterior view

Together the quadriceps are known as "The Four Faced Trouble maker".

VASTUS MEDIALIS
"BUCKLING KNEE MUSCLE"

PAIN PATTERN

- Medial/anterior knee pain
- Deep ache in knee
- Radiation up to lower/medial thigh
- Localized pain

SYMPTOMS

- Minimal limited ROM
- Knee buckles inward
- Unexpected weakness without atrophy (muscle suddenly feels weak)

CAUSATIVE/PERPETUATING FACTORS

- Sedentary lifestyle
- Chronic kneeling
- Hyperextension of knee
- Sudden overload through misstep or fall
- Sudden stopping with a twist
- Improper lifting/squatting – knees in
- Knee surgery
- Hiking/running downhill
- Excessively tight hamstrings
- Excessive pronation of foot – lower compartment

CORRECTIVE ACTIONS

- Quad stretch
- Knee flexion

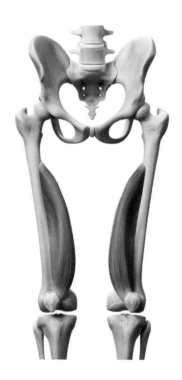

Anterior view

VASTUS INTERMEDIUS
"THE FRUSTRATER"

PAIN PATTERN

- Front of the thigh – most intense at mid-thigh

CAUSATIVE/PERPETUATING FACTORS

- Sedentary lifestyle
- Chronic kneeling
- Hyperextension of knee
- Sudden overload through misstep or fall
- Sudden stopping with a twist
- Improper lifting/squatting
- Knee surgery
- Hiking/running downhill
- Excessively tight hamstrings
- ACL tear

CORRECTIVE ACTIONS

- Quad stretch
- Knee flexion

Trigger points in vastus intermedius are typically secondary to developed trigger points in other quad muscles.

SYMPTOMS

- Difficulty straightening leg
- Difficulty standing from seated position
- Difficulty using stairs

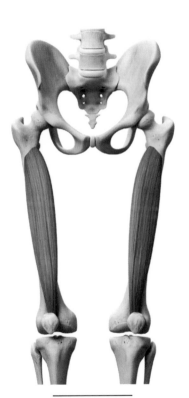

Anterior view

VASTUS LATERALIS
"STUCK PATELLA MUSCLE"
"NEST OF HORNETS"

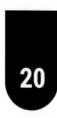

PAIN PATTERN

- Trigger points around lateral aspect of thigh (localized pain)
- "Nest of hornets" most common at knee
- Lateral thigh pain
- Posterior aspect of knee
- Crest of ilium

SYMPTOMS

- Patella locks into place (limited ROM)
- Pain around lateral patella
- Difficulty lying on side

> Vastus Lateralis is the most common quad to develop trigger points.

CAUSATIVE/PERPETUATING FACTORS

- Sedentary lifestyle
- Chronic kneeling
- Hyperextension of knee
- Sudden overload through misstep or fall
- Sudden stopping with a twist
- Improper lifting/squatting
- Knee surgery
- Hiking/running downhill
- Excessively tight hamstrings
- Overload during eccentric contraction
- Side to side motions – skiing, slack lining, balance beam

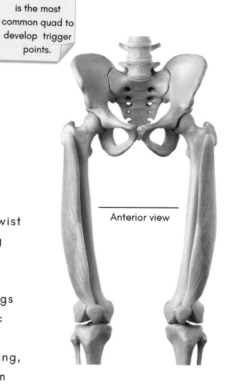

Anterior view

CORRECTIVE ACTIONS

- Check for trigger points in glute minimus
- Quad stretch
- Knee flexion

CORRECTIVE ACTIONS (CONT.)

- Cross client's affected leg over the other, pull leg towards unaffected side

TENSOR FASCIAE LATAE
"PSEUDO-TROCHANTERIC BURSITIS"

PAIN PATTERN

- Anterolateral pain over greater trochanter
- Pain deep in hip, down lateral aspect of thigh, to knee

CAUSATIVE/PERPETUATING FACTORS

- Walking/running on uneven surfaces
- Hiking, hurdles, getting into high cars
- Lunges
- Sudden fall or misstep
- Immobilization of limb
- Hip surgery
- Lower compartment dysfunction (bow legs, etc.)

CORRECTIVE ACTIONS

- Cross client's affected leg over the other, pull leg towards unaffected side
- Side lunge
- Avoid lotus, butterfly stretch
- Avoid sitting cross-legged
- Bent-knee cross-body stretch
- Foam roller
- Tennis ball against wall

SYMPTOMS

- Pain may feel like trochanteric bursitis
- Prevents walking rapidly or lying comfortably on affected side
- Affects gait
- Difficulty and pain sitting with hip fully flexed
- Difficulty lying on side without pillow between knees

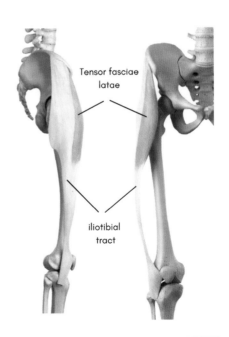

Tensor fasciae latae

iliotibial tract

Lateral view of right hip & thigh

Anterior view of right hip & thigh

SARTORIUS
N/A

PAIN PATTERN

- Trigger points and pain through entirety of muscle
- Localized pain

CAUSATIVE/PERPETUATING FACTORS

- Trigger points in associated musculature (TFL is a secondary muscle)
- Sudden stopping/twisting
- Chronic hip flexion
- Improper gait
- Near fall or misstep

CORRECTIVE ACTIONS

- Compression with stretching
- Foam roller
- Avoid butterfly/lotus

SYMPTOMS

- Superficial tingling
- No positional or stretching relief
- No limited ROM

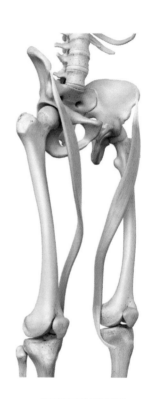

Lateral, anterior, & medial view of hip & thigh

Treat Sartorius thoroughly. Trigger points are often latent and can be activated by partial treatment.

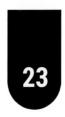

ADDUCTORS (MAGNUS, LONGUS, BREVIS)

"OBVIOUS PROBLEM MAKERS"

23

PAIN PATTERN

Longus/Brevis:
- Trigger points project pain proximally and distally
- Upper/medial part of knee extending down to tibia
- Deep in groin/pelvis

Magnus:
- Up into groin below inguinal ligament
- Down thigh nearly to knee
- May be difficult to have bowel movement
- Deep pain
- "Generalized internal pelvic pain"
- "Pain shooting up into pelvis and exploding like fireworks"

CAUSATIVE/PERPETUATING FACTORS

- Sex
- Sudden overload
- Osteoarthritis of hip/hip surgery
- Running uphill or downhill
- Sitting for a long period of time
- Crossing legs while sitting

Longus:
- Horseback riding

Magnus:
- Skiing

CORRECTIVE ACTIONS

- Avoid extended shortening of adductors/hip flexion (sitting for long periods)

SYMPTOMS

Longus/Brevis:
- Pain in groin and medial thigh during activity
- Made worse when weight-bearing and sudden twist of hip

Magnus:
- Intra-pelvic pain - localized to vagina, rectum and deep within the pelvis
- Difficulty positioning lower leg (when side-lying)

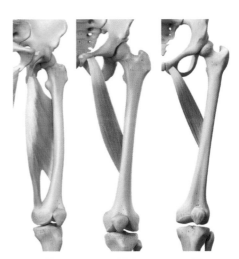

Adductor Magnus	**Adductor Longus**	**Adductor Brevis**
Medial and anterior view of left hip & thigh	Anterior view of left hip & thigh	Anterior view of left hip & thigh

CORRECTIVE ACTIONS (CONT.)

- Regular application of moist heat
- Stretch - standing with spread legs, shift hips side to side

PECTINEUS
"THE FOURTH ADDUCTOR"

PAIN PATTERN

- Deep, local groin pain just below inguinal ligament
- May also project pain to upper part of anterior thigh
- Hip joint
- May extend to pubic tubercle

SYMPTOMS

- Related muscles are usually involved
- Limited abduction of hip

CAUSATIVE/PERPETUATING FACTORS

- Fall/near fall
- Sex
- Sudden overload
- Osteoarthritis of hip/hip surgery/fracture of neck of femur
- Running uphill or downhill
- Sitting for a long period of time
- Crossing legs while sitting (jackknife position, sitting on one leg)
- Horseback riding

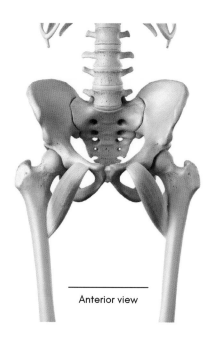

Anterior view

CORRECTIVE ACTIONS

- Avoid extended shortening of adductors/hip flexion (sitting for long periods of time)
- Regular application of moist heat

CORRECTIVE ACTIONS (CONT.)

- Stretch – standing with spread legs, shift hips side to side

GRACILIS
N/A

PAIN PATTERN

- Superficial pain along inside of thigh
- Hot, stinging pain

CAUSATIVE/PERPETUATING FACTORS

- Overload in other adductor muscles
- Misstep/fall

CORRECTIVE ACTIONS

- Walking
- Avoid extended shortening of adductors/hip flexion (sitting for long periods of time)
- Regular application of moist heat
- Correct functional leg length discrepancy
- Stretch - standing with spread legs, shift hips side to side
- Place pillow between knees when sleeping/side-lying

SYMPTOMS

- Pain at rest

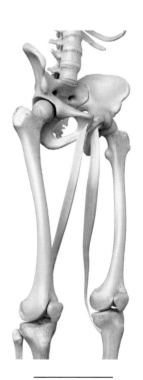

Lateral, anterior & medial view

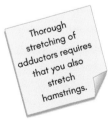

Thorough stretching of adductors requires that you also stretch hamstrings.

ILIOPSOAS
"THE HIDDEN PRANKSTER"

PAIN PATTERN

- Along the spine ipsilaterally from thoracic region to sacroiliac (sometimes to upper buttock)
- Anterior thigh and groin pain associated with certain movements
- Pain may spill over to sacrum, back, anterior thigh

CAUSATIVE/PERPETUATING FACTORS

- TrPs activated secondarily/simultaneously with other muscles group
- Sudden fall
- Prolonged sitting
- Placing knees higher than hips
- Sleeping in fetal position
- Tightness is rectus femoris

CORRECTIVE ACTIONS

- Routinely perform hip extending exercising
- Sit back and sit up exercise

The iliopsoas is contraindicated for the entire duration of pregnancy.

SYMPTOMS

- "Throwing out" back
- Difficulty pooping /constipation
- Lower back pain (vertically down spine)
- Pain is worse when patient stands up right from bent or seated position
- Nagging back pain when recumbent
- Pain in front of thigh
- Difficulty standing from deep seated chair
- Inability to do sit-ups
- Unable to straighten back while standing

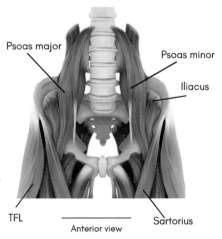

Psoas major

Psoas minor

Iliacus

TFL

Anterior view

Sartorius

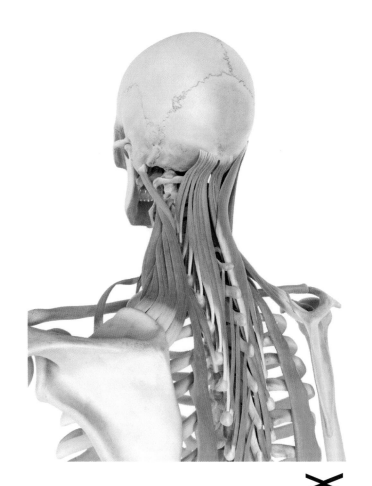

SPINE & THORAX

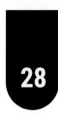

RECTUS ABDOMINIS + THE ABDOMINALS

THE LIMBO LIMITERS

Abdominals: external oblique, internal oblique, transversus abdominis.

PAIN PATTERN

Rectus abdominis:

- TrPs at attachment site
- Horizontal PP across lower back and midback
- Lower right quadrant
- Sub umbilical TrP

Others:

- Referred pain in the same quadrant of the back
- Urinary, bladder, sphincter spasms
- Mimics appendicitis

CAUSATIVE/PERPETUATING FACTORS

Rectus abdominis

- Poor posture
- Visceral disease
- Direct trauma
- Emotional stress
- Vomiting
- Scar tissue
- Over exercise
- Constipation

Others:

- Stress
- Poor posture
- Vigorous sports/activity
- Coughing
- Chronic twisted position

SYMPTOMS

Rectus abdominis:

- Dysmenorrhea (painful period)
- Nausea, heartburn, indigestion, upset stomach, diarrhea, anal leakage, projectile vomiting, belching, acid reflux/gird
- Painful bowel movements

Others:

- Amenorrhea (lack of period)

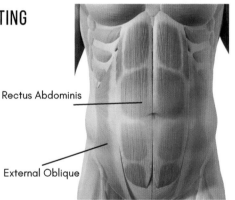

Rectus Abdominis

External Oblique

Anterior view

CORRECTIVE ACTIONS

- Small pillow for lumbar support
- Wearing loose, comfortable belts/pants
- Abdominal/diaphragmatic breathing
- Stretch (cobra)

ERECTOR SPINAE
N/A

PAIN PATTERN

Iliocostalis thoracis:
- Pain in thoracic region of back (Sometimes abdomen)
- Restriction of spinal motion

Iliocostalis lumborum:
- Pain referred downward
- Low in buttock
- Along iliac crest

Longissimus thoracis:
- Pain is referred low in buttock

Multifidi/Rotatores:
- Hurts at the attachment sight

SYMPTOMS

- Iliocostalis can cause breast pain
- "Lumbago"
- Chief complaint is lower back and sometimes the buttock pain
- Steady ache, deep in the side
- Client is convinced pain is from spine
- Muscles will become inflamed
- Difficulty bending to pick things up

CAUSATIVE/PERPETUATING FACTORS

- Poor posture
- Improper lifting techniques
- Sudden overload or sustained/repeated muscular contraction
- Sitting with a wallet in back pocket
- Change in gait
- Whiplash
- Prolonged immobility

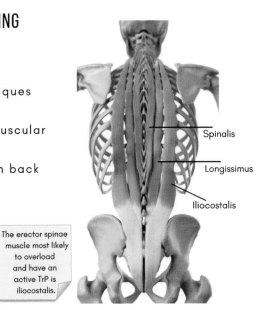

The erector spinae muscle most likely to overload and have an active TrP is iliocostalis.

Spinalis

Longissimus

Iliocostalis

Posterior view

CORRECTIVE ACTIONS

- Stretching
- Proper lifting techniques
- Moist heat/hot bath
- Leg traction (one at a time)

SERRATUS POSTERIOR SUPERIOR/INFERIOR

30

N/A

> Overloads with forward head posture and disrupted breathing patterns.

PAIN PATTERN

Superior:
- Deep, sharp pain under scapula
- Pain down elbow, front and back of the wrist, ulna side of hand (front and back), pinky finger

Inferior:
- Type 1 TrP (hurts where it is)
- Aching discomfort over and around muscle
- Pain in lower back

CAUSATIVE/PERPETUATING FACTORS

Superior:
- Overload in the trapezius
- Side lying
- Posture, coughing, paradoxical breathing (asthma, anxiety), upper respiratory ailment
- Lifting heavy objects
- Sitting for long periods

Inferior:
- Strain through a combined movement of lifting, turning, and reaching
- Hyper extended reach over head

SYMPTOMS

Superior:
- Pain while side lying
- Deep ache under scapula
- Pain in forearm, hand, and entire pinky finger
- Occasionally pectoralis pain
- Numbness in hand
- Steady to deep ache at rest

Inferior:
- Guarded, shallow breathes
- Sharp pain in back when coughing
- Nagging ache in lower thoracic region

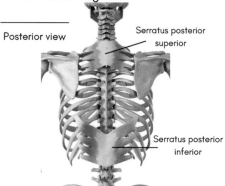

Posterior view — Serratus posterior superior — Serratus posterior inferior

CORRECTIVE ACTIONS

- ROM neck stretches
- Correct postural abnormalities
- Add lumbar support to back of chair
- Breath work exercises

QUADRATUS LUMBORUM

"THE JOKER OF THE LOW BACK PAIN"
"HIP HIKER"

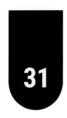

PAIN PATTERN

- Lateral border of the iliac crest
- Over the greater trochanter
- Lower abdomen (similar PP to
- psoas)
- Outer aspect of lower thigh
- Sacroiliac joint
- Deep within the center of the
- buttock
- Groin, anterior thigh, testicles/scrotum

SYMPTOMS

- Unable to stand upright
- Difficulty walking
- Aching low back pain
- Leg length discrepancy
- Inability to turn over in bed
- Disrupted sleep
- Prevented weigh baring on same side – hip "goes out"
- Pain down leg from QL to lower leg

CAUSATIVE/PERPETUATING FACTORS

- Overload by simultaneously bending and lifting
- Improper lifting
- Sustained and repetitive strain
- Sudden [imposed] leg length discrepancy (use of ankle cast/boot)
- Near fall

CORRECTIVE ACTIONS

Client may to crawl into office if QL is overloaded, due to inability to stand upright and weight bare.

- Ice application
- Stretch
- Remove wallet from back pocket while sitting
- Correct leg length differential
- Side sleeping with upper leg on pillow

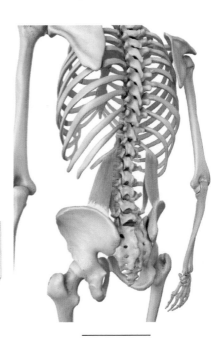

Lateral, posterior & medial view

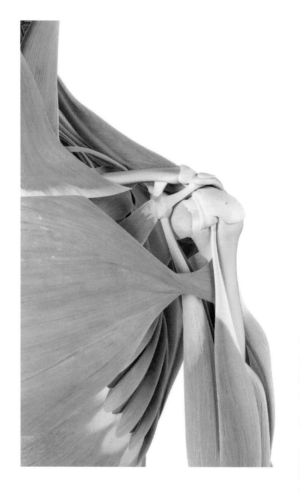

SHOULDER & ARM

PECTORALIS MAJOR
"CHEST AND SHOULDER NUISANCE"

PAIN PATTERN

- Anterior aspect of shoulder
- Anterior deltoid region
- Anterior chest and breast
- Extend down ulnar arm to forth and fifth digits
- PP referred unilaterally (hurts where it is)
- Pain in clavicular section
- Most active TrP are in the axillary junction point

CAUSATIVE/PERPETUATING FACTORS

- Overload from heavy lifting
- Immobilization of the arm in adducted position (sling or cast)
- Sustained rounded shoulder position
- Sustained anxiety levels
- Poor posture
- Prolonged sitting
- Visceral effects from heart attack

CORRECTIVE ACTIONS

- In-doorway stretch exercises with 3 arm position

SYMPTOMS

- Pain in elbow
- Numbness in forth and fifth digits
- Pain in half of the third digit
- Chest pain
- Breast tenderness with hyper sensitivity of the nipple
- Intrascapular back pain (from rounded shoulders)
- Downward and forward pull of medial clavicle
- Restricted abduction (particularly horizontally)
- Difficulty wearing a bra or shirt

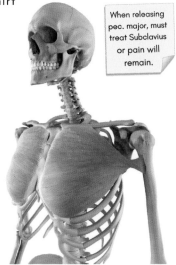

When releasing pec. major, must treat Subclavius or pain will remain.

Medial, anterior and lateral view

PECTORALIS MINOR
"THORACIC OUTLET IMPOSTER"

PAIN PATTERN

- Referred to eight different muscles
- Upward to sub clavicular area
- Entire pectoral region to the same side
- Down ulnar section arm, elbow, forearm and last three fingers

SYMPTOMS

- No distinction between pectoralis major
- Limitations reaching forward and up or reaching backward with arm at shoulder level
- Restricted ROM
- Numbness, tingling, pain down arm

CAUSATIVE/PERPETUATING FACTORS

- Forward-leading posture
- Compression from backpack straps
- Kickback from shotgun
- Satellite TrP due to myocardial ischemia or pectoralis major
- Whiplash
- Strain or over use
- Crutches

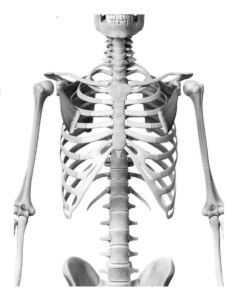

Anterior view

CORRECTIVE ACTIONS

- Doorway stretch exercises with three arm position

SERRATUS ANTERIOR
"STITCH IN SIDE MUSCLE"

PAIN PATTERN

- Anterolateral aspect of the chest
- Medial inferior angle of the scapula
- Radiation down ulnar surface of homolateral arm and may extend as far as the palm and ring finger
- Persistent, intense pain

CAUSATIVE/PERPETUATING FACTORS

- Fast or prolonged running
- Push-ups
- Overhead lifting
- Chin-ups
- Severe coughing

CORRECTIVE ACTIONS

- Stretching

SYMPTOMS

- "Air hunger" – can't take a deep enough breath
- Sharp pain when TrP is touched or breath is increased
- Hurts to do any kind of workouts
- Shortness of breath
- Cannot find a comfortable position
- Collapsed posture due to pain
- Unable to lie on affected slide
- Unable to finish ordinary sentence without shortness of breath

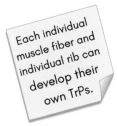

Each individual muscle fiber and individual rib can develop their own TrPs.

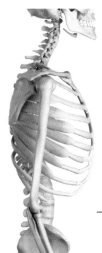

Lateral view

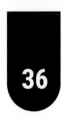
SUPRASPINATUS
"OVERHEAD ACTIVITY ARCH ENEMY"

PAIN PATTERN

- Middle of the deltoid region
- Downward over arm and forearm
- Lateral epicondyle (AKA tennis elbow)
- Rarely extends to wrist

CAUSATIVE/PERPETUATING FACTORS

- Carrying heavy objects (suitcase, briefcase)
- Walking large dogs that pull on leash
- Lifting an object to or above shoulder
- Prolonged abducted posture (hair stylists)

CORRECTIVE ACTIONS

- Avoid carrying heavy objects
- Avoid sustained contraction of muscles
- Avoid lifting heavy object over head
- Stretching- pull forearm across and upward behind the back, pull with other arm
- Pull arm across chest with other arm
- Stretch on a stool while sitting a warm shower

SYMPTOMS

- Deep ache when arm is at rest
- Pain during abduction
- Difficulty reaching above shoulder
- Painful "catch" when reaching up – must change posture to complete movement
- Pain at night that disturbs sleep
- Dull ache at rest
- Stiffness in shoulder

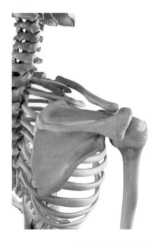

Referred pain in the rotator cuffs can activate satellite TrPs.

Posterior and lateral view of right shoulder

INFRASPINATUS
"SIDE-SLEEPER'S NEMESIS"

PAIN PATTERN

- Base of the skull on the same side
- Deep in the deltoid region and shoulder joint
- Extends down the front of the lateral aspects of the arm and forearm
- Radial half of hand
- Occasionally pain in the fingers
- Between spine and scapula
- Vertebral border of scapula

CAUSATIVE/PERPETUATING FACTORS

- Overload while reaching backwards and upwards
- Pulling or carrying heavy weight
- Acute stress/overload; chronic stress/overload
- Tennis
- Car accident
- Bracing yourself when falling

CORRECTIVE ACTIONS

- Application of hot pack/moist hear for 10-15
- TrP compression by laying on a tennis ball (or using Theracane) for 1-2 minutes EOD

SYMPTOMS

- Headaches
- Pain sleeping on either side and sometimes on the back
- Unable to reach behind back
- Inability to brush teeth or hair
- Pain in the front of the shoulder (deep within the joint)
- Difficulty putting effected arm in coat jacket
- Inability to medially rotate and abduct the arm
- Weakness of grip (dropsies)
- Loss of mobility at the shoulder

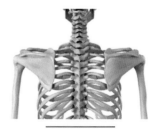

Posterior view

CORRECTIVE ACTIONS (CONT.)

- Sleep while hugging a pillow
- Self-stretching
- Slow, deep breaths will allow gravity to release pressure

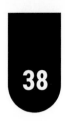

TERES MINOR

"INFRASPINATUS LITTLE BROTHER"
"THROWER'S TRIAL"

PAIN PATTERN

- Pain in the distal deltoid
- Posterolateral arm
- Sharp/deep pain persists even after infraspinatus worked out
- Mimics bursitis

SYMPTOMS

- Posterior shoulder pain
- Radiculopathy of forth and fifth fingers
- Difficulty reaching back
- Painful bursae
- Pain in back of shoulder

CAUSATIVE/PERPETUATING FACTORS

- Repetitive medial and laterally rotation of arm
- Overload of muscle by reaching up and behind the shoulder
- Overload of infraspinatus
- Motor vehicle accident
- Volleyball

CORRECTIVE ACTIONS

- Hang from a bar
- Avoidance of excessive or repetitive overload of the muscles
- Avoid lying on effect arm while asleep
- Apply moist heat
- TrP pressure release daily (tennis ball/ Theracane)
- Hot pack and ROM will complete the Tx

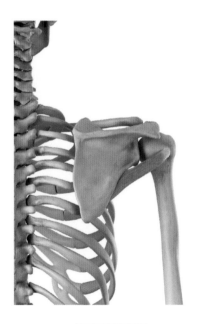

Posterior view of
the right shoulder

SUBSCAPULARIS
"PSEUDO FROZEN SHOULDER SYNDROME"

PAIN PATTERN

- Posterior shoulder down the triceps area of the elbow - skips and shows up as a band around the wrist
- Posterior deltoid over scapula and down lateral arm

CAUSATIVE/PERPETUATING FACTORS

- Repetitive external/internal rotation
- Swimming
- Pitching a baseball
- Kettlebell swings
- Sudden shoulder trauma
- Stress on the shoulder joint
- Prolonged immobilization of the shoulder joint in the adducted or medial rotation (using a sling)
- Rounded shoulder posture

CORRECTIVE ACTIONS

- When sleeping on painful side - keep a small pillow between elbow and side of chest
- Correction of postural stress
- Stretch arm when sitting for long period of times

SYMPTOMS

- Discomfort while wearing a watch
- Pain down the arm without inhibiting reach
- Pain at rest and at motion
- Restriction of abduction
- Inability to reach across to opposite armpit

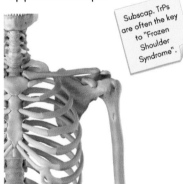

Subscap. TrPs are often the key to "Frozen Shoulder Syndrome".

Anterior view of the left shoulder

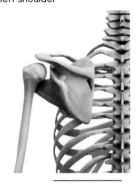

Posterior view of the left shoulder

LATISSIMUS DORSI
"MIDBACK MANIPULATOR"

PAIN PATTERN

- Inferior area of scapula and surrounding midthoracic region
- Back of shoulder
- Down medial aspect of arm, forearm, and hand including ring and middle finger
- Affects the Traps, erector spinae, triceps and wrist extensors
- Front of shoulder, lower lateral aspect of trunk, above iliac crest

CAUSATIVE/PERPETUATING FACTORS

- Lifting/holding/pulling down heavy objects over head
- Acute trauma or overload (blunt force trauma or injections)
- Consistent compression (bra band)
- Throwing a basketball
- Crutches

CORRECTIVE ACTIONS

- Stretch - grab wrists above head, pull wrist on affected side to opposite side
- Doorway stretch exercise (a few reps daily)

SYMPTOMS

- Back ache unresponsive to stretch or position change
- Pain while reaching out forward and up to lift something bulky
- Unable to identify cause
- Most active back, hip, arm pain while sleeping
- Inability to lie comfortably
- Disrupted sleep
- Difficulty wearing a bra
- Midthoracic myofascial pain

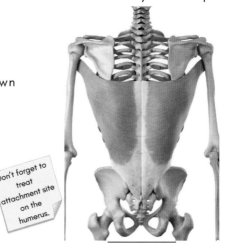

Don't forget to treat attachment site on the humerus.

Posterior view

CORRECTIVE ACTIONS (CONT.)

- Moist heat
- TrP pressure release using a tennis ball with arm extended over the head

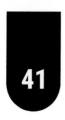

TERES MAJOR

"LAT'S LITTLE BROTHER"
"FORGOTTEN SHOULDER AGITATOR"

PAIN PATTERN

- Posterior deltoid region
- May refer pain into shoulder joint posteriorly
- Occasionally to dorsal forearm
- Extend to extensor surface of the forearm

CAUSATIVE/PERPETUATING FACTORS

- Depressor movements that overload
- Pulling something down from above
- Holding heavy, bulky objects
- Local injections on trigger point

CORRECTIVE ACTIONS

- Doorway stretch
- Inactivation of satellite TrP

Muscle Test:
reach both hands
over head, lower
hand has
restricted teres
major.

SYMPTOMS

- Difficulty abducting the arm and placing it against homolateral ear
- Shoulder pain when reaching forward and up (serving a tennis ball)
- Little restriction in motion
- Pain in motion is the main complaint

ALWAYS treat with latissimus dorsi.

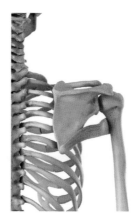

Posterior view of
right shoulder

RHOMBOIDS
"SHOULDER BLADE SORCERERS"

PAIN PATTERN

- Concentrates along medial border of the scapula
- May extend laterally over supraspinous area of the scapula
- Hurts where it is (intrascapular pain)

CAUSATIVE/PERPETUATING FACTORS

- Lifting, pushing, pulling
- Holding your arms above your head for long periods of time (styling hair)
- Rounded shoulder posture
- Hyper tonic PECS

CORRECTIVE ACTIONS

- Stretches
- Correct posture while seated (desk work/driving)
- Theracane/tennis ball TrP therapy
- Treat pectoralis muscles
- Stimulate/strengthen the back muscles
- Doorway stretches

SYMPTOMS

- Local, superficial, aching pain while at rest and not influenced by movement
- Snapping/crunching feeling during movement of scapula
- No limited ROM

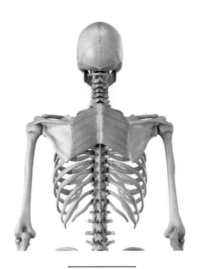

Posterior view

Satellite PPs can be caused by TrP in levator or trapezius.

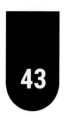
DELTOID

"OVERT BOTHERED"

PAIN PATTERN

Anterior Fibers:
- Anterior and medial deltoid
- Weakened abduction of externally rotated arm

Posterior Fibers:
- Posterior and medial deltoid
- Weakened abduction of internally rotated arm

CAUSATIVE/PERPETUATING FACTORS

- Overexertion
- Sudden overload
- Impact trauma (blunt force trauma or injections)
- Overloaded supraspinatus
- Prolonged lifting or holding at shoulder height
- Repetitive, vigorous, jerky motion (mowing the lawn, hedge trimming, walking a large dog)

CORRECTIVE ACTIONS

- Doorway stretch (anterior and middle fibers)
- Pull arm forward and push on elbow towards opposite side (posterior fibers)
- Daily passive stretching
- Treat/inactivate any TrP that are referring pain to deltoids

SYMPTOMS

- Muscle fatigue
- Shoulder pain
- Pain on shoulder motion (less frequent at rest)
- Difficulty bringing hand to mouth or reaching back
- Inability to reach 90° of abduction
- Painful "catch" at 15° of elevation
- Popping and cracking when moving shoulder (combination of supraspinatus/deltoid overload)

Repeated overuse can cause microtraumas in the muscle.

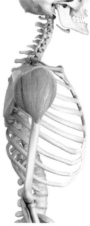

Lateral view of right shoulder

BICEPS BRACHII
N/A

PAIN PATTERN

- Type I TrP (hurts where it is)
- Upward over biceps area and front of shoulder
- Bicipital aponeurosis
- Bicipital groove (biceps tendon)
- Some spill over to supraspinous

CAUSATIVE/PERPETUATING FACTORS

- Overstressed during activity
- Back hand motion during tennis/ping pong/disc golf/baseball
- Manually using a screw driver
- Satellite TrP from infraspinatus overload
- Carrying heavy loads

CORRECTIVE ACTIONS

- Press the tendon in the groove and move the arm slowly (active release)
- Against the door jam exercise: thumb up/arm extended, turn your body away: repeat with thumb down
- Lift things with hand pronated instead of supinated

SYMPTOMS

- Weight of a jacket hurts shoulder
- Superficial anterior shoulder pain
- Pain during elevation of arm above the shoulder during flexion and abduction
- Weakness/pain when raising pain above head
- Snapping sounds from the long tendon during abduction of the arm
- Soreness in upper trapezius region
- Arm "catches" when raising the arm

Tx the biceps and triceps together because they're antagonistic.

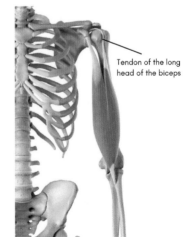

Tendon of the long head of the biceps

Anterior view of left shoulder and arm

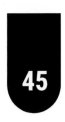

BRACHIALIS
"BEER DRINKER'S MUSCLE"

45

PAIN PATTERN

- Base of the thumb on palmar and dorsal side
- TrP just above the antecubital area (above elbow)

CAUSATIVE/PERPETUATING FACTORS

- Secondary to radial nerve entrapment
- Continuing overload of forearm flexion
- Carrying heavy weight
- Compression of bicep area of the arm while it's fully extended (sleeping on your arm while arm is extended)

CORRECTIVE ACTIONS

- Lifting only light or moderate loads with arm supinated
- Place a pillow in the angle of the elbow while sleeping
- Avoid carrying purse/heavy bags on forearm
- Active release techniques

SYMPTOMS

- Tingling, numbness in base of thumb

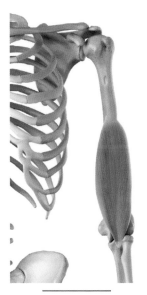

Anterior view of left shoulder and arm

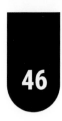

CORACOBRACHIALIS
"ARMPIT MUSCLE"

PAIN PATTERN

- Anterior aspect of proximal humerus
- Interrupted patter of pain that extend back of arm, forearm and back of hand (skips elbow and wrist)
- Disabling pain and restricted ROM

CAUSATIVE/PERPETUATING FACTORS

- Does not overload on itself: overloads due to muscles in functional unit (pec. major, biceps brachii, deltoid anterior)

CORRECTIVE ACTIONS

- Avoid lifting heavy objects with arms outstretched in front (keep elbows close to body)
- Doorway stretch in lower hand position (daily)
- Moist heat before or after passive stretch exercises

SYMPTOMS

- Inability to reach into back pocket
- Difficulty reaching back to put arm in jacket
- Upper limb pain
- Pain shows up AFTER treating muscles in functional unit

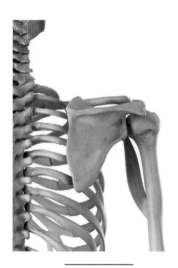

Posterior view of right arm

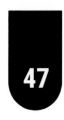

TRICEPS BRACHII
N/A

PAIN PATTERN

- Posterior arm
- Lateral condyle
- Spill over to forth and fifth finger
- Upper part of suprascapular region

CAUSATIVE/PERPETUATING FACTORS

- Overload stress (pushing/pulling heavy objects)
- Rapid extension of the forearm
- Pulling a heavy object
- Golf; push-ups; manual transmission; tennis; walking a dog; carrying heavy objects with your elbow bent
- Walking with crutches/a cane

CORRECTIVE ACTIONS

- Stretching
- Elbow support while driving; sitting in a chair; working on a computer
- Properly size crutches/cane
- Reduce weight of tennis racket or objects being carried

SYMPTOMS

- Inability to straighten arm to ear with arm above head
- Elbow, forearm, hand pain

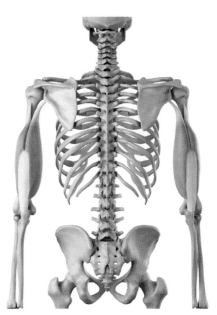

Posterior view

Triceps brachii is the only extender of the elbow.

It is also the only prime mover muscle that crosses two joints.

ANCONEUS
N/A

PAIN PATTERN

- Refers pain to lateral epicondyle
- Olecranon process

CAUSATIVE/PERPETUATING FACTORS

- Overloaded triceps

CORRECTIVE ACTIONS

- Tx triceps

> The anconeus muscle fulfills the same tasks at the elbow as the triceps muscle

SYMPTOMS

- Cannot lean on elbow or put elbow down without pain

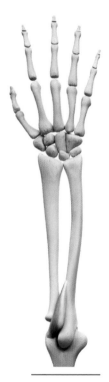

Posterior view of right elbow and hand

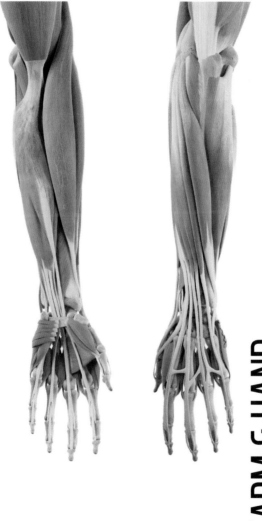

FOREARM & HAND

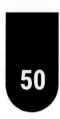

SUPINATOR
"THE TENNIS ELBOW MUSCLE"

PAIN PATTERN

- Lateral epicondyle
- Elbow
- Dorsal web of thumb
- Sometimes – lateral antecubital area

SYMPTOMS

- Elbow pain at rest and while carrying heavy object
- Elbow "jerks" when pouring beverages

CAUSATIVE/PERPETUATING FACTORS

- Carrying heavy briefcase; opening a stiff doorknob; walking a dog with elbow fully extended; opening tight jar lids
- Back hand strokes (tennis)
- Resisting unexpected pronation
- Forceful elbow flexion while arm is pronated

CORRECTIVE ACTIONS

- Discontinue lifting/supinating
- Carry heavier objects supinated and not pronated
- Stretching
- Strength training

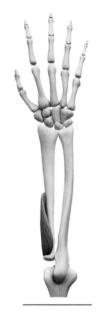

Posterior view of right elbow and hand

Forearm muscles in order of palpation:
- Extensor Carpi Radialis
- Extensor Carpi Digitorum
- Extensor Carpi Ulnaris
- Supinator
- Brachioradialis (dividing the extensors from the flexors on radial side)
- Flexor Carpi Radialis
- Flexor Carpi Ulnaris
- Pronator Teres
- Extensor digitorum

PRONATOR TERES
N/A

PAIN PATTERN

- Deep in volar radial region of wrist and forearm
- Some spill over pain to thumb

CAUSATIVE/PERPETUATING FACTORS

- Fracture at wrist or elbow
- Use of a cane

CORRECTIVE ACTIONS

- Stretch
  - Extend the arm out, pronate, pull fingers back
  - Relax shoulders, with hands in a prayer position rotate hands to point at the ground (without altering your shoulders)

Carpal tunnel syndrome will impinge median nerve between bones.

SYMPTOMS

- Unable to supinate cupped hand (like receiving change)
- Trigger finger (inability to straighten) in the thumb
- Radiculopathy to palm of hand and volar area of wrist (due to restriction of the medial nerve)

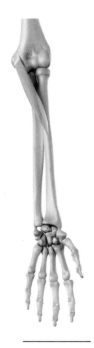

Anterior view of left forearm and hand

BRACHIORADIALIS
N/A

PAIN PATTERN

- Lateral epicondyle
- Down length of muscle
- Web of the thumb
- Dorsal aspect of hand

SYMPTOMS

- "Tennis elbow"
- Unreliable or weak grip

CAUSATIVE/PERPETUATING FACTORS

- Overuse of gripping/twisting motion
- Gardening
- Using a screw driver
- Knitting/crochet

CORRECTIVE ACTIONS

- Stretch
- Rest the muscles

Brachioradialis divides the extensors from the flexors on radial side.

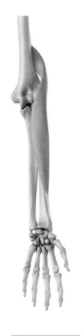

Anterior view of left forearm and hand

EXTENSORS OF THE FOREARM + WRIST

N/A

PAIN PATTERN

- Lateral epicondyle
- Lightly over dorsal aspect of forearm
- Dorsal side of hand
- Dorsal side of wrist

CAUSATIVE/PERPETUATING FACTORS

- Overworked hands
- Satellite TrPs caused active TrP
- Opening tight jars
- Extensive hand shaking
- Excessive typing
- Disc golf/frisbee

CORRECTIVE ACTIONS

- Avoid forceful activity while deviating the hand
- Stretch
  o Full extension of elbow then extend wrist

PPs could also be satellite TrPs of main muscles in the shoulder and upper arm.

SYMPTOMS

- Pain in the back of the arm, hand, and wrist
- Weakness of grip when deviating wrist
- Inhibition of muscles (they quit/"dropsies")
- "Writer's cramp"

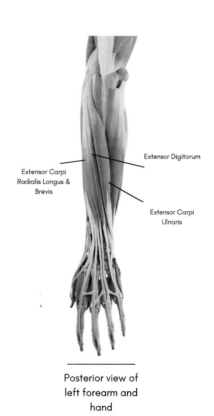

Extensor Digitorum

Extensor Carpi Radialis Longus & Brevis

Extensor Carpi Ulnaris

Posterior view of left forearm and hand

FLEXORS OF THE FOREARM + WRIST

N/A

PAIN PATTERN

- Throughout length of digit
- Pain extends like lightening beyond the digit
- Pain centers on volar (inside) wrist crease

CAUSATIVE/PERPETUATING FACTORS

- Repetitive or prolonged strong gripping
- Twisting or pulling motions of the hand and fingers
- Unsupported elbow at rest
- Satellite TrP from pectoralis minor, latissimus dorsi, or serratus posterior superior
- Stretching the extensors
- Walking with a cane

CORRECTIVE ACTIONS

- Compress and friction tendons at knuckles
- Moist heat
- Support the elbow, arm, wrist, and hand while at rest
- Massaging the carpals, joints, and interosseous tissue
- Finger flutter exercise ("dead hand" shake)
- Stretch
  - Extend elbow, flex wrist

SYMPTOMS

- "Trigger finger" pain
- Pain while using scissors/shears
- Pain while cupping and supinating hand (receiving change)
- Difficulty putting a clasp in hair
- Inability to supinate hand and extend arm
- "Weeder's thumb"

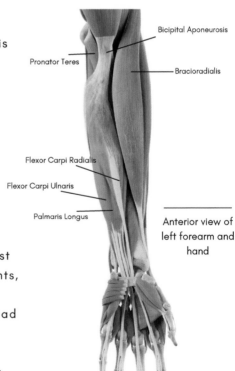

Bicipital Aponeurosis
Pronator Teres
Bracioradialis
Flexor Carpi Radialis
Flexor Carpi Ulnaris
Palmaris Longus

Anterior view of left forearm and hand

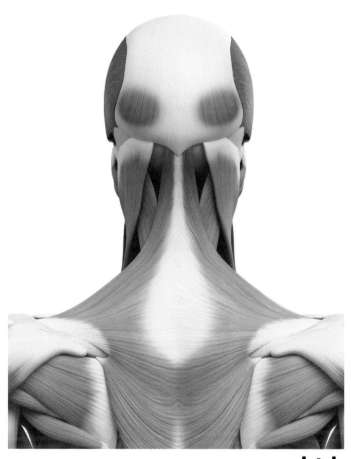

HEAD, NECK, FACE

TRAPEZIUS
"THE STRESS HEADACHE PRODUCER"

PAIN PATTERN

Upper fibers:
- Posterolateral aspect of the neck, behind ear, temple

Middle fibers:
- Pain toward vertebrae, posterior shoulder

Lower fibers:
- Refer pain to neck, suprascapular and intrascapular regions
- Little restriction to ROM
- Anterior aspect of the neck to the clavicle
- Refer pain unilaterally

CAUSATIVE/PERPETUATING FACTORS

- Sustained lateral flexion of the head and neck
- Elevation of the shoulders
- Compression of upper shoulders
- Whiplash

CORRECTIVE ACTIONS

- Theracane/tennis ball TrP compression
- Stretching
- Improve work ergonomics
- Avoid shoulder compressions with heavy backpack/purse

SYMPTOMS

Upper fibers:
- Tension headache around temple/behind eyes
- Goosebumps or "shivers" up and down spine
- Lower molar teeth
- Occiput pain/tension
- Angle of jaw/"TMJ" pain

Middle Fibers:
- Superficial burning over rhomboids
- Achy pain on top of shoulder and acromion
- Goosebumps ipsilateral triceps area

Lower Fibers:
- Refers up to cervical and suprascapular region

Most common muscle in the body to develop TrP.

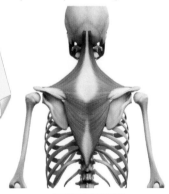

Posterior view

LEVATOR SCAPULAE
"CRICK IN THE NECK"

PAIN PATTERN

- Pain in the angle of the neck and posterior aspect of the shoulder and midscapular region
- Limited ROM to affected side

CAUSATIVE/PERPETUATING FACTORS

- Sustained rotation of the head and neck to one side
- Emotional tension
- Coughing
- Elevated shoulders
- Whiplash
- Backpack/bra/purse compressions
- Forward head posture

SYMPTOMS

- Pain in back of neck
- "Stiff neck"
- DROM
- Mechanical neck pain (painful movement)
- Inability to turn head to affected side
- Pain radiates down to supramedial border of scapular

Most common TrP is at insertion of scapula.

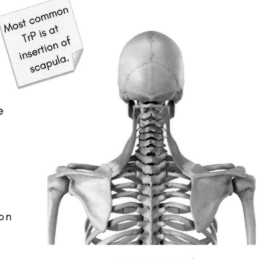

Posterior view

CORRECTIVE ACTIONS

- Stretching
- Postural correction
- Proper sleeping position (better pillows)
- Heat application
- Theracane/tennis ball TrP therapy
- Improved desk ergonomics
- Treat pectoral muscles

SPLENII -
SPLENIUS CAPITIS + SPLENIUS CERVICIS
N/A

PAIN PATTERN

Splenius Capitis:
- Pain at the top of the head (dome/cap of pain)

Splenius Cervicis:
- Ache inside the skull
- [Sometimes] downwards and inside the shoulder girdle and the angle of the neck

CAUSATIVE/PERPETUATING FACTORS

- Forward head posture
- Pregnancy posture
- Look up for long periods of time (installing garage doors/painting ceilings/ construction work)
- Leaning with your hand on your chin will overload muscles bilaterally
- Whiplash/impact trauma
- Rapid stretch/rapid contraction

CORRECTIVE ACTIONS

- Cold packs
- Self-stretch exercise
  - Roll head from side to side
  - Tilt head from side to side
  - Look up and look down

SYMPTOMS

- Both splenii overloaded unilaterally will cause a homolateral blurring of vision
- Slightly stiff neck (minor DROM)
- Dizziness when standing up from seated or lying position
- Vertigo

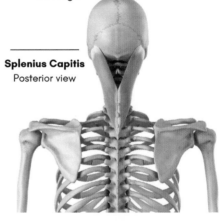

Splenius Capitis
Posterior view

Stiffness in the neck from the splenii will not be as prominent as levator scapula.

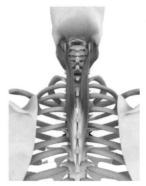

Splenius Cervicis
Posterior view

SUBOCCIPITALS
"THE BOBBLE HEAD MUSCLES"
"GHOSTLY HEADACHE MUSCLES"

PAIN PATTERN

- Headache unilaterally from occiput to eye
- Pain deep inside the skull and hard to localize
- Pain blurs with other posterior cervical muscles

SYMPTOMS

- Headache when pressure applied to back of head (pillow at night)
- Inability to turn head (checking blind spots while driving)

CAUSATIVE/PERPETUATING FACTORS

- Propping head on elbows
- Excessive anterior head position or forward head posture
- Sustained head flexion
- Looking to one side for extended periods of time
- Holding a phone to your ear with your shoulder
- Whiplash

CORRECTIVE ACTIONS

- Passive self-stretches
- Avoid sustained upward gaze
- Keep back of the neck warm
- Avoid leaning forward while working on a computer or reading

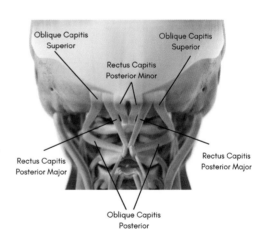

Oblique Capitis Superior

Oblique Capitis Superior

Rectus Capitis Posterior Minor

Rectus Capitis Posterior Major

Rectus Capitis Posterior Major

Oblique Capitis Posterior

Posterior view

Rectus capitis major & minor are "yes" muscles.

Obliqui Inferior & Superior are "no" muscles.

STERNOCLEIDOMASTOID (SCM)

N/A

PAIN PATTERN

- Pain referred to frontal area, extends across the forehead to the opposite side
- Homolateral deep ear pain
- Cheek, temple, and orbit pain
- Arches of the cheeks
- Scalp tenderness

CAUSATIVE/PERPETUATING FACTORS

- Whiplash/sidelash – MVA
- Forward head posture
- Chronic rotation to one side
- Compression of the neck (tight tie/tight collars)
- Chronic cough or paradoxical breathing
- Tight pec major putting tension on SCM

CORRECTIVE ACTIONS

- Self-massage
- Posture correction
- Stretching
- Avoid prolonged turning of the neck

The SCM is one of the only muscles that refers pain to the other side.

SYMPTOMS

- Tears/redness of the eye
- Visible head tilt to one side
- Ringing in the ears
- Unilateral deafness
- Tension headaches
- Vertigo
- Ipsilateral sweating (same
- side as TrP)
- Blurred or double vision
- Dry cough
- Sore throat/lump in throat
- Cheek and molar pain on same side
- Difficulty breathing while sleeping on back

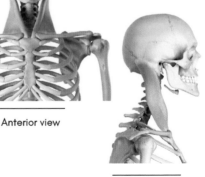

Anterior view

Lateral view

SCALENES- ANTERIOR, MIDDLE, POSTERIOR

N/A

PAIN PATTERN

- Persistent, aching pain
- Radiates downward toward chest
- Laterally to the upper arm
- Pain skips elbow and reappears at radial side of forearm, hand, thumb, and index finger
- Radiates posteriorly into midscapular area

CAUSATIVE/PERPETUATING FACTORS

- Whiplash/sidelash – MVA
- Forward head posture
- Paradoxical breathing/ chronic cough
- Chronic rotation of the cervical spine
- Pulling/lifting/tugging
- Medial rotation of the arms
- Compression from T-back bras
- Breast reduction

CORRECTIVE ACTIONS

- Stretches
- Breath work
- Posture correction
- Correction of poor posture
- Proper body mechanics

SYMPTOMS

- Headaches
- Puffiness in pinky and ring finger
- Pain to medial border of the scapula

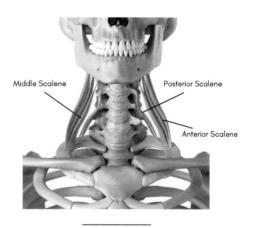

Middle Scalene   Posterior Scalene

Anterior Scalene

Anterior view

Anterior scalene when over-loaded will entrap the nerves/blood flow that supply the arm.

DIGASTRIC
"PSEUDO SCM PAIN"

PAIN PATTERN

- Lower angle of the jaw
- Four bottom front teeth
- Area of the chin below the four front teeth
- Pain referred to the tongue
- TrP extends to the ear

SYMPTOMS

- Difficulty swallowing
- Feeling of a lump in the throat that won't go down
- Headaches

CAUSATIVE/PERPETUATING FACTORS

- Whiplash – MVA
- Forward head posture
- Tight neck fascia
- Tight abdominals/pectoral region
- Bruxism
- Misalignment of the teeth

CORRECTIVE ACTIONS

- Myofascial release anterior neck and chest, as well as, abdomen (pin & post)
- Lean forward with chin rest on hand – with other hand, move hyoid bone back and forth
- If jaw deviates when opening the mouth – use counter resistance (press jaw back in line while opening mouth)

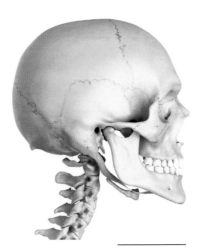

Lateral view

Digastric refers pain bilaterally no matter which side of the body has the TrP.

ALL OTHER ANTERIOR NECK MUSCLES

PAIN PATTERN

- Referred pain to the tongue
- Laryngeal region
- Anterior neck
- Mouth region
- Elevated first rib

CAUSATIVE/PERPETUATING FACTORS

- Whiplash - MVA
- Forward head tilt
- Unresolved posterior neck pain
- Tight neck fascia
- Tight abdominals/pectoral region
- Bruxism
- Misalignment of the teeth

CORRECTIVE ACTIONS

- Myofascial release anterior neck and chest, as well as, abdomen (pin &post)
- Lean forward with chin rest on hand - with other hand, move hyoid bone back and forth
- Correct teeth misalignment

SYMPTOMS

- Difficulty swallowing/lump in
- the throat
- Pain while talking
- Sore throat with no infection/redness
- Numbness/tingling/ inflammation in arm and hand (due to compression from elevated first rib)
- Dry mouth
- Persistent tickle in the throat
- Reoccurring or chronic hoarse voice
- Pain under the tongue when talking/eating (mylohyoid TrP)
- Mouth watering all the time (mylohyoid TrP)

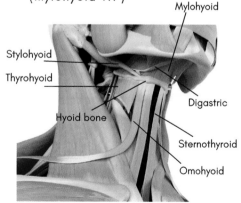

Mylohyoid
Stylohyoid
Thyrohyoid
Hyoid bone
Digastric
Sternothyroid
Omohyoid

Lateral, anterior
and medial view

MUSCLES OF THE FACE

TEMPORALIS

PAIN PATTERN

- Temporal headache
- Homolateral maxillary toothache (upper teeth)
- Temporal region to eyebrow

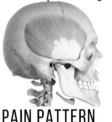

Temporalis
Lateral View

SYMPTOMS

- Headache
- Teeth sensitivity to heat/cold
- Feeling of "loose" tooth
- Restricted jaw movement
- Crooked smile
- Inability to open mouth
- Face pain

MASSETER

PAIN PATTERN

- Pain in upper teeth and cheek
- Sinus pain
- Pain in lower teeth and jaw
- Pain above eyebrow

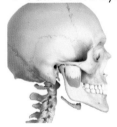

Masseter
Lateral View

SYMPTOMS

- Ringing in homolateral ear (if bilateral ringing occurs—symptoms are caused by something else)
- Restricted mouth opening with deviation to ipsilateral side
- Sensitivity to heat/cold
- Face Pain

PTERYGOIDS

The pterygoid muscles are located in the infratemporal fossa of the skull.

PAIN PATTERN

- Generalized pain in mouth and TMJ region
- Vague ache in back of the mouth
- Behind the jaw joint and deep in the ear

SYMPTOMS

- Sore Throat
- Difficulty swallowing
- Painful/restricted jaw opening
- Clicking of the jaw
- Stuffiness/echoing in the ear

MUSCLES OF THE HUMAN BODY

ABDOMINALS	28
ADDUCTOR GROUP	
Adductors	23
Gracilis	25
Pectineus	24
ANCONEUS	48
ANTERIOR NECK MUSCLES	
Digastric	62
Scalenes	61
Sternocleidomastoid	60
Other	63
BICEPS BRACHII	44
BRACHIALIS	45
BRACHIORADIALIS	52
CORACOBRACHIALIS	46
DELTOID	43
ERECTOR SPINAE GROUP	29
EXTENSORS OF THE ANKLE + TOES	
Extensor Digitorum Longus / Extensor Hallicus Longus	09
EXTENSORS OF THE FOREARM + WRIST	53
FLEXORS OF THE FOREARM + WRIST	54
FLEXORS OF TOES	05
GASTROCNEMIUS	02
GLUTEALS	
Gluteus Maximus	13
Gluteus Medius	14
Gluteus Minimus	15
HAMSTRINGS	
Biceps Femoris	11
Semitendinosus/ Semimembranosus	12
ILIOPSOAS	26
LATERAL ROTATORS OF THE HIP	16
LATISSIMUS DORSI	40
LEVATOR SCAPULAE	57
MASSETER	64
PECTORALIS MAJOR	33
PECTORALIS MINOR	34
PERONEUS LONGUS/BREVIS	08
PIRIFORMIS	16
POPLITEUS	06
PRONATOR TERES	51
PTERYGOIDS	64
QUADRATUS LUMBORUM	31
QUADRICEP MUSCLES	
Rectus Femoris	17
Vastus Intermedius	19
Vastus Lateralis	20
Vastus Medialis	38
RHOMBOIDS	42
ROTATOR CUFF MUSCLES	
Infraspinatus	37
Subscapularis	39
Supraspinatus	36
Teres Minor	38

INDEX

SARTORIUS	22
SERRATUS ANTERIOR	35
SERRATUS POSTERIOR SUPERIOR/INFERIOR	30
SOLEUS	03
SPLENII	58
SUBOCCIPITALS	59
SUPINATOR	55
TEMPORALIS	64
TENSOR FASCIAE LATAE	21
TERES MAJOR	41
TIBIALIS ANTERIOR	07
TIBIALIS POSTERIOR	04
TRAPEZIUS	56
TRICEPS BRACHII	47

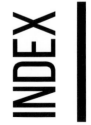

INDEX

Travell, Janet, and David Simmons. *Myofascial Pain and Dysfunction: The Trigger Point Manual*, vol. I Baltimore: Williams and Wilkins, 1983.

Travell, Janet, and David Simmons. *Myofascial Pain and Dysfunction: The Trigger Point Manual*, vol. II Baltimore: Williams and Wilkins, 1992.

Finando, Donna, and Steve Finando. *Trigger Point Therapy for Myofascial Pain*. Rochester, Vermont: Healing Arts Press, 2005

Biel, Andrew. *Trail Guide to the Body*. Fifth Edition. Boulder, CO: Books of Discovery, 2014

BIBLIOGRAPHY

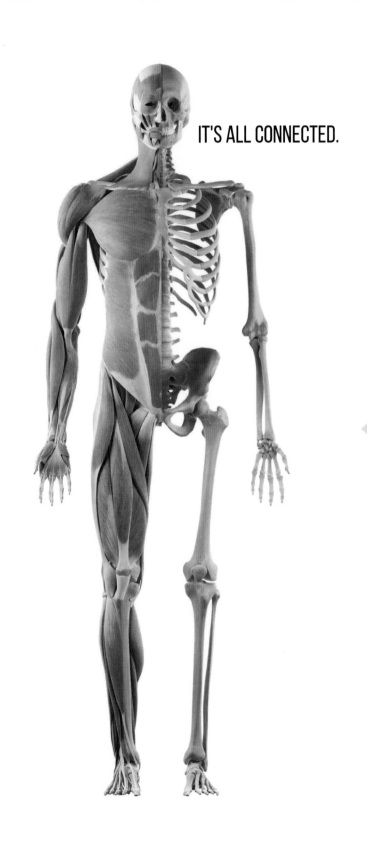

IT'S ALL CONNECTED.

Printed in Great Britain
by Amazon

64661375R00043